THE BLEEDING ECOSYSTEM

Promoting Regenerative Agricultural Techniques

BY

Robert Lawrence

TABLE OF CONTENTS

INTRODUCTION

Regenerative farming approach focuses on restoring soils that have been degraded by overuse or too much exposure to artificial fertilizers and pesticides through industrial and agricultural practices. Conversely, regenerative farming's methods promote conservation and healthier ecosystems by rebuilding soil's organic matter through holistic farming and grazing techniques.

The agriculture industry currently ranks as one of the largest emitters of carbon dioxide in the world. Combined with deforestation and poor forest management, it makes up a third of all man-made greenhouse emissions. Globally, people, and industries, are becoming increasingly interested in adopting sustainable practices, and within agriculture, there is considerable pressure to reduce emissions and limit waste.

It describes farming and grazing practices that aim at reversing climate change by rebuilding soil organic matter and restoring degraded soil biodiversity – resulting in both carbon drawdown and improving the water cycle. Regenerative agriculture encourages us to think about how all aspects of agriculture are connected through a network of entities who grow, enhance, exchange, distribute, and consume goods and services—instead of a linear supply chain. It embodies farming and ranching in a style that nourishes people and the earth, with specific practices varying from farmer to farmer and from region to region.

HISTORY OF REGENRATIVE AGRICULTURE

Robert Rodale coined the term "regenerative organic" to describe a holistic approach to farming that encourages continuous innovation and improvement of environmental, social, and economic measures. The number one priority in regenerative organic agriculture is soil health.

Soil health is intrinsically linked to the total health of our food system. The health of the soil affects everything from plant health to human wellbeing and the future of our planet.

Regenerative agriculture prioritizes soil health while simultaneously encompassing high standards for animal welfare and worker fairness. The idea behind this farming system was to create farm systems that work in harmony with nature to improve quality of life for everybody involved.

The core principles behind the dynamic system of regenerative agriculture are basically to restore soil and ecosystem health, address inequity, and leave our land, waters, and climate in better shape for future generations. The regenerative agriculture movement is the dawning realization among more people that an Indigenous approach to agriculture can help restore ecologies, fight climate change, rebuild relationships, spark economic development, and bring joy.

IMPORTANCE OF REGENERATIVE AGRICULTURE

The care and creativity regenerative farmers showcase yield benefits on and off the land. They grow food and fiber, draw down carbon, conserve water, replenish waterways, grow healthier foods, reduce their use of synthetic inputs, employ people within their communities, and ensure the long-term vitality of the land.

The loss of the world's fertile soil and biodiversity, along with the loss of indigenous seeds and knowledge, pose a deadly threat to our future survival. According to soil scientists, at current rates of soil destruction, we will not only suffer serious damage to public health due to a qualitatively degraded food supply characterized by diminished nutrition and loss of important trace minerals, but we will literally no longer have enough arable topsoil to feed ourselves. Without protecting and regenerating the soil on our vast acres of cultivated farmland, pastureland, and forest land, it will be impossible to feed the world, keep global warming below 2 degrees Celsius, or halt the loss of biodiversity.

We need to realize that working landscapes provide not just products but also ecosystem services like carbon sinks, water recharge, and evolutionary potential. We need agriculture that does not lose our carbon and does not deplete our people. By contrast, the industrial agricultural system that dominates Western food and fiber supply chains encourages practices that promote soil erosion at a rate of 10 to 100 times higher than soil formation; nutrient runoff and harmful algal blooms in freshwater and coastal systems; and monocropping and other threats to local biodiversity, including critical pollinators. These systems compartmentalize natural resources and focus on the yields of individual crops.

ECOLOGICAL BENEFITS OF REGENERATIVE AGRICULTURE

IMPROVEMENTS IN SOIL HEALTH AND FERTILITY
While the techniques for caring for the soil vary with the context of each farm, generally, regenerative growers limit mechanical soil disturbance. Instead, they feed and preserve the biological structures that bacteria, fungi, and other soil microbes build underground—which provide above-ground benefits in return.

In cases of extreme weather and climate change, it has been observed that yields on farms practicing regenerative agriculture are significantly higher than conventional farms.

REDUCE RELIANCE ON SYNTHETIC INPUTS
Regenerative agriculture practitioners make every effort to reduce their reliance on synthetic inputs, such as herbicides, pesticides, and chemical fertilizers. In the process of prioritizing soil health, majority of them naturally use fewer chemical inputs. Instead, as beneficial insects and wildlife return and diverse crop and livestock rotations disrupt weed cycles, the ecosystem becomes more resilient. And with fewer toxic chemicals, there are reduced human health risks as well as increased financial independence through cost savings from reduced use of these synthetic inputs. A pesticide- and artificial fertilizer-free environment is healthier as it does not expose you or your farm workers to toxic synthetic agricultural chemicals. Prolonged exposure to pesticides has been linked to a higher prevalence of neurological diseases. The greater your exposure to chemicals, the more likely you are to suffer from a variety of health problems ranging from headaches and fatigue to memory loss.

Similarly, studies have identified the huge potential that exists in converting food by-products from cities into regenerative soil enhancers that are comparable or even better than synthetic fertilizers. Companies like SoilFood in Finland and Lystek in Canada are proving that this is possible in reality.

NURTURE COMMUNITIES AND PROMOTE LOCAL ECONOMIES

Many regenerative farmers begin their practice with the aim of growing healthy food for their families and communities. They consider it essential to treat their farmworkers, apprentices, and other laborers with respect, and to provide on-farm staff with fair wages and a seat at the decision-making table. And many of these growers have a deep appreciation of the social and historical contexts in which they operate. They acknowledge how unjust policies have shaped American agriculture, even though our food systems were built by Black and Indigenous communities. This system of family farming presents an opportunity to boost local economies.

INCREASE FOOD PRODUCTION AND PRESERVE AGRICULTURAL LAND

Considering that by the year 2050 we will need to feed a world population estimated to be about 10 billion, farms and ranches need to make even greater efforts to sustainably increase their productivity. Of course, as population increases, farmland is impacted in different ways in different regions. In some places, agricultural land is at risk of conversion to suburban and urban development. According to American Farmland Trust, 2,000 acres of agricultural land are converted by development every day in the United States. Supporting regenerative farms and ranches that embrace crop and animal diversity while boosting yields can help farms stay in business and prevent farmland from being lost to other uses.

In other areas, mainly in tropical and subtropical regions, forests and grasslands are being converted for agricultural uses. Farmland isn't just increasing in these places but it's also shifting into more ecologically fragile areas, which are vital for healthy ecosystems. Land management efforts that complement regenerative agriculture practices would help to preserve these natural carbon sinks along with wildlife habitat and biodiversity. Abandoned or unproductive farm and ranch lands should be reforested or restored to natural ecosystems to minimize further land degradation and soil erosion.

In the 21st-century conventional agriculture incurs other indirect costs that cannot be ignored. The long-term threat of climate change to the natural environment is well established, and agriculture bears much of the responsibility for this. It has been established that 23% of the total global greenhouse gas (GHG) emissions are directly related to "agriculture, forestry and other types of land use". Conversely, regenerative agriculture seeks to increase the organic matter in the soil, which makes it better able to sequester carbon from the atmosphere, meaning it has the potential to reduce climate change instead of contributing to it.

Regenerative farming is friendlier to the climate because it stores carbon in healthy soil, and reduces energy requirements by relying more on physical and animal labor rather than fossil fuels. It eliminates the use of petroleum-based fertilizers and pesticides and supports natural ecosystems that store carbon, such as forests and prairies. Lastly, it reduces the production of greenhouse gases due to a reduction in fossil fuel use.

What actually constitutes a healthy soil or ecosystem? How can we easily measure it so we know that farms are on the right trajectory? US organizations such as the Nature Conservancy and the Soil Health Institution are now working with tech companies to use remote sensing and soil modeling to come up with new methods of measuring soil health over large landscapes.

INFILTRATION AND BIODIVERSITY

Regenerative farming has other demonstrable benefits besides improving soil health and helping to fight climate change. Improving the soil not only increases fertility in a sustainable way but also tends to improve water infiltration. Better infiltration means less runoff, and also less erosion and pollution from the soil being carried away in the runoff water. In some areas, water springs that dried up several years ago have begun to flow again due to new regenerative farming approaches.

An increase in biodiversity also tends to make ecosystems more sustainable and resilient. Regenerative agriculture focuses more attention on the quality of life and growth on a farm.

Although climate change has increasingly entered the mainstream consciousness, yet another environmental disaster, the drastic depletion of agrobiodiversity, quietly threatens the global food supply. Agro-biodiversity is the various biological entities that contribute to food growing, encompassing the numerous plant varieties, animals and microorganisms which support functions of agro-ecosystems.

Since the beginning of food production there have been a large variety of food crops, however, a mere twelve crops make up 80 percent of the global plant-based dietary energy. Only four crops – wheat, rice, maize and potato – provide approximately 60 percent of plant-derived protein and calories.

Aside from depending on a limited number of crops, the food system worldwide still depends on a small genetic makeup. High-yielding and genetically standardized varieties have superseded 70% of the world's maize from conventional varieties, in addition to 50% of the wheat in Asia, Africa, and Latin America; and 75%

of rice in Asia. Diversifying production and creating a space for biodiversity in agriculture, as the indigenous have been doing for centuries, is incredibly important in the face of climate change.

PROMOTES MIXED FARMING SYSTEM

Regenerative agriculture allows for integration on the same farming unit or for partnerships with neighboring livestock businesses. There are opportunities for grazing cover crops and for short- to medium-term grass or herbal leys. With livestock comes manure, which returns varying levels of nutrients and organic matter to the soil, reducing the need for manufactured fertilizer.

REGENERATIVE AGRICULTURE TECHNIQUES

The key to regenerative agriculture is that it improves the land using technologies that regenerate and revitalize the soil and the environment. Regenerative agriculture leads to healthy soil, capable of producing high quality, nutrient dense food while simultaneously improving, rather than degrading land, and ultimately leading to productive farms and healthy communities and economies. It is a dynamic and holistic, incorporating permaculture and organic farming practices, including conservation tillage, cover crops, crop rotation, composting, mobile animal shelters and pasture cropping, to increase food production, farmers' income and especially, topsoil.

There are many practices that falls under the regenerative agriculture system which vary from one farmer to another.

Cover cropping: The practice of planting crops in soil that would normally otherwise be bare after a cash crop is grown and harvested. By keeping living roots in the soil, cover crops reduce soil erosion, increase water retention, improve soil health, increase biodiversity, and more. They can be planted during harvest time or in between rows of permanent crops.

Intensive rotational grazing: An Indigenous practice that mimics the way large animals moved in herds across grasslands. This method of grazing moves livestock between pastures on a regular basis to improve soil fertility and allow pasture grasses time to regrow.

No-till farming: A technique that leaves the soil intact when planting rather than disturbing the soil through plowing.

Composting: The natural process of turning waste from manure or food into fertilizer.

Reduced or no fossil fuel–based inputs: Building soil health and leveraging other natural systems to help manage pests and reduce the reliance on pesticides or other chemicals, regardless of whether a farmer decides to pursue organic certification.

Agroforestry: An Indigenous practice wherein growers mimic forest systems by integrating trees and shrubs into crop and animal systems.

EFFECT OF REGENERATIVE AGRICULTURE ON CLIMATE CHANGE

Agriculture plays a significant role in contributing to climate change. Our food systems are also suffering enormous consequences from rising temperatures and increases in extreme weather events like droughts and floods.

This system of agriculture addresses the climate crisis with practices that sequester more carbon in the soil and help make farmland—and local communities—more resilient. In fact, farming and ranching can play an important part in natural climate solutions, as described below.

Soil is one of the earth's greatest carbon sinks, thanks to photosynthesis and microbes. With proper care, soil can draw down 250 million metric tons of carbon dioxide–equivalent greenhouse gasses every year—and that's just in the United States.

It Boosts Climate Resilience
As flood, drought, and other extreme weather patterns become more frequent, farmers and ranchers are preparing their land to be more resilient. Healthy soils with high amounts of organic matter are able to absorb more water during a flood—to the benefit of the farmer and downstream communities—and even help maintain water security during a drought. Ranchers can also help prevent wildfires by grazing livestock to control bush.

Eradicate Fossil Fuels from Agriculture
Our climate and health depend on ending our reliance on fossil fuel–based fertilizers and pesticides. Farmworkers and their

communities are in constant danger of exposure to these chemicals, putting them at risk of suffering acute and chronic health issues.

Reduce Greenhouse Gas Emissions in Agriculture
A study conducted by U.S. Environmental Protection Agency showed that about 10 percent of U.S. greenhouse gas emissions are attributed to farming and ranching, with the largest sources being livestock (such as cows), agricultural soils, and rice production. Some regenerative practices—including no-till farming, cover cropping, and rotational grazing—can decrease overall emissions from the agricultural sector.

HOW TO SUPPORT REGENERATIVE AGRICULTURE

Encouraging Investments in Regenerative Agriculture
Despite all the benefits of regenerative agriculture, only a small percentage of U.S. farms have adopted regenerative practices—in part because U.S. farm policy does not prioritize them. But some states have started to encourage farmers, ranchers, and private landowners to adopt practices that reduce greenhouse gas emissions. In California, there are incentive programs like the Healthy Soils Initiative, the Biologically Integrated Farming Systems Program, and Sustainable Agriculture Lands Conservation Program. Since 2017, Iowa's Department of Agriculture has been offering a $5-per-acre "good farmer discount" on crop insurance premiums to farmers who plant cover crops. These types of initiatives can serve as a model for other states looking to reward farmers for better management. Incentivizing these practices is only the first step toward transformative, systemic agricultural change. In addition, by directing technical assistance and financial resources to Black, Latino, and Indigenous farmers and other disadvantaged growers, we can begin to address historic injustices in our food system.

Part of what's needed now is a more holistic policy platform—one that pushes for transformational changes to our food and fiber system alongside the grassroots organizations, community leaders, artists, and revolutionary farmers we are learning from

Promoting Regenerative Agriculture at Home
We can join the regenerative agriculture movement by demanding proper stewardship of our land through regenerative agriculture. Talking to our neighbors and local policymakers and supporting organizations that are trying to build better soil.

A knowledge of who grows your food, how they grow it, and where it's grown is a crucial step toward building regenerative food systems and shortening our agricultural supply chain. This can be achieved in the grocery store or supermarket by asking the store owner what they know about the food they source. Connection with the local farmers at a farmers' market or farm visit also helps.

Composting at home: Divert your household food waste from the landfill while closing the loop of our nutrient-and-soil cycle.

Be a regenerative agriculture consumer: Know how your food is sourced and choose meat, dairy, and produce that are grown to help regenerate land. When dining out, opt for restaurants that source ingredients from regenerative farmers.

Grow your own food: Follow regenerative agriculture techniques no matter what size your plot is. Feel empowered to start your own regenerative garden.

REGENERATIVE FARMING VERSUS ORGANIC FARMING

It is commonly accepted that organic farming produce are grown without the use of pesticides, synthetic fertilizers, sewage sludge, genetically modified organisms, or ionizing radiation. Animals that produce meat, poultry, eggs, and dairy products are not given antibiotics or growth hormones.

In a sense, organic farming is about a return to farming's roots. Up until the 20th century, all food was produced "organically." With the industrialization of the agriculture sector, synthetic fertilizer, chemical pest-control practices, and Genetically Modified Organisms(GMO) were introduced to increase productivity.

It was only in the 1940s a counter-movement arose that reframed the farm as an organism, requiring a holistic, ecologically balanced approach to farming. This is not a knock-on organic farming. At the time organic farming methods were gaining popularity in the mid-20th-century, the focus of many environmentalists was very much about reducing the harm inflicted on the environment. By that measure, it works. Organic farming does reduce the harm to the environment.

It is quite telling that the EU is hoping to convert one-quarter of agricultural land to be "managed organically" by 2030. The EU's rationale is that organic farming is better suited to protecting biodiversity by reducing the reliance on pesticides in particular. This target now forms part of the European Green Deal and the Farm to Fork strategy.

But as things stand in the 21st century, the world is approaching the limits of what it can handle, and agriculture needs to not just reduce the damage it inflicts, but actually heal the land, without compounding any other global issues.

That's where regenerative agriculture comes into play, It's growing food and agricultural products in a way that mimics nature. Moving from extracting nutrients and minerals from the soil… to increasing the biology in the field and building soils.

Like organic farming, regenerative agriculture is a loosely defined set of concepts that can vary depending on where you look, but ultimately it seeks to reverse negative impacts rather than eliminate them. This can only be realized if regenerative agriculture is looked at as a landscape management exercise that aims to increase local biodiversity, increase soil fertility, empower local communities, and fundamentally try to farm in nature's form."

Many of these regenerative solutions overlap with and build on the principles of organic farming to make sure that soils are being actively restored.

Leaving land dormant between cash-crop seasons qualifies as organic farming, but some practitioners go the extra mile through pioneering solutions that also qualify as regenerative, such as by applying diverse cover crop mixes to increase organic matter and soil biology, produce natural fertilizer, and reduce erosion.

Regenerating the biology in the soil using techniques such as cover cropping also helps sequester carbon, addressing the challenge of climate change while simultaneously preserving nutrients in the soil.

A study comparing regenerative cultivation of corn in the United States versus conventional farming approaches found that although the yield was 29% lower, the regenerative farms were 78% more profitable because farmers did not have to spend as much on their operations. That is because regenerative agriculture requires fewer external inputs such as fertilizer due to improved soil organic matter.

Unlike organic farming, which leans towards the traditional, regenerative agriculture is also faster to adopt 21st-century solutions. Sensor technology can help farmers practice precision cultivation, while satellite crop health imagery can allow farmers to examine crop health at each growing stage and to map out fixed trails for transport to conduct tillage, crop care, and harvesting — minimizing soil load and preserving soil structure on the majority of the land.

With the right combination of techniques, the total farm yield can even be maintained by improving biodiversity on-farm through measures such as adding wildlife habitat to farmland, reducing soil tillage, and enriching soil with organic matter.

BARRIERS TO REGENERATIVE AGRICULTURE

It's a lifestyle choice now which is a barrier to really scaling it up. But organic farming is a good starting place to build on.

If the food system needs to become regenerative, what are the barriers? While some techniques such as cover cropping are generally agreed to be part of "regenerative agriculture," the definition remains murky, and many other beneficial practices are in a grey area. Organic farming may not have a specific definition, but certifications at least provide for a clear understanding of what the required practices are.

Regenerative farming is an ideal, but it is missing the concrete structures that could bring it to life: legal definitions, certifications, and clear methods of measurement and monitoring.

On the one hand, regenerative farming is a combination of individual practices like agroforestry, intercropping, and minimal soil disturbance. Making it a reality would then be a matter of integrating these techniques, one farm at a time. On the other hand, perhaps the definition should be ingrained in the goals of regenerative farming: to rehabilitate the soils and improve above-ground biodiversity.

A major challenge relates to implementation. At small scales, the transition from conventional to regenerative can be quite short with little investment required. However, at a large scale, the change can take much longer, creating periods of uncertainty in an already low-margin sector. In the case of Leontino Balbo's 16,000-hectare sugar cane farm, it took 27 years to achieve the full transformation. The reasons for this vary. They can be biological, as building soil organic matter and a healthy population of soil microbes happens over many seasons. Other obstacles are business-oriented. New equipment may need to be purchased; farm activities and schedules redesigned; staff to be retrained, and new scientific knowledge to be acquired.

Alleviating the risks associated with this transition period is where governments or the financial sector could play a role, by offering subsidies, incentives, or some other kind of insurance. To enable this support, we will need new ways of monitoring progress.

DISADVANTAGES OF REGENERATIVE AGRICULTURE

In integrating different elements on the farm, the regenerative farmer seeks to revive the classic mixed-farm model, which is an important consideration in the post-COVID food industry. By producing a greater diversity of foodstuffs on one site, a farm can reduce external inputs and outputs, and thus reduce the risk of contamination.

However, to practice regenerative agriculture effectively, many farmers will need to acquire new knowledge and skills, particularly in respect of soil management. And managing farmers' expectations of results might be difficult, as critics have accused exponents of over-claiming on yield and benefits. By not tilling the soil, farmers can save between 30 and 40 percent of the time and can decrease the amount of soil erosion in certain terrains, but the disadvantages of regenerative agriculture are, in many cases, that more unwelcome plants grow on the land, and some farmers compensate for this by increasing their use of the herbicide.

And it is possible that the extent of soil degradation is exaggerated too. The degradation of soils is difficult to measure, and there are huge variations between estimates by different bodies.

Public consciousness regarding sustainability in agriculture still has a long way to go in this region. Governments are slow to offer farm subsidies to encourage the implementation of regenerative agricultural practices. Without this additional support and encouragement from official sources, it is difficult to grow specialized products in a market saturated with commodity products. Consequently, you are left taking more risks that leave you financially vulnerable.

Regenerative agriculture requires more work to produce goods that are ready for sale. There is more physical burden like pulling weeds and other cultivation techniques, which in conventional agriculture can be dealt with using artificial pesticides and tillage machines.

Requires specialized knowledge
The quality of a crop produced through regenerative farming is heavily reliant on your skills, knowledge, and experience. In regenerative farming, you have to monitor crop growth patterns during every critical stage of growth. If you are unable to recognize and address a problem, the value of the crop may be affected. You also need in-depth local knowledge about soil systems, ecology, meteorology, and other factors that can influence the growth of crops.

Unique marketing challenges
Most farmers like yourself will agree that organic foods are more expensive than commodity foods or commercially grown products. Currently, the local market for organic foods is not as defined as it is for other crops. This makes it difficult for specialty farmers to compete with other commercially produced products that are available easily at lower costs.

Rigorous certification process
To be certified as an organic producer, you need to spend more money to hire certifying agents, which adds to the overall cost of production.

Initial high cost than commercial farming
In order to qualify as a regenerative farming enterprise, you need to invest in infrastructure and other start-up costs. Soil amendments, such as rock dust, are more expensive for many farmers when compared to the chemicals traditionally used in commodity farming.

Reduced profit margins and increased costs
Any new agricultural system that doesn't incorporate conventional methodologies will require larger initial investments and work. This means that you may have reduced profit margins. It takes time. Trees do not grow overnight and soil needs time to improve. It takes planning and organization. A long-term plan is a must. The setup can be labor-intensive.

REGENERATIVE FARMING AND THE FUTURE OF FOOD SUSTENANCE

Sustainable by definition means that something is able to be maintained at a certain rate or level. Which is all fine and well until you consider the world, we currently live in. About 38% of global agricultural land is already affected by degradation. So "sustainable" isn't going to cut it anymore, we need to regenerate. 'Sustainability is a bridge – regeneration is the destination' Regenerative agricultural practices or techniques are similar to that of sustainable agriculture, but the tools and techniques are customized to the specific agroecosystem in which it takes place and is soil-based rather than seed based. Attention is given to increasing the amount of nutrients cycling through soil by improving soil organic matter while also increasing the soil's potential for storing carbon. All in all, regenerative agriculture aims at regenerating, renewing and further improving the soil functions and capabilities for ecosystem services in an always-improving process. We focus on regenerative because we do not want to simply sustain the current state of the world's soil. That would be almost like going to the doctor for a sickness and he said he could make it so you couldn't get any sicker, you just wouldn't ever be better. The same thing is happening now, our soil is sick and we need to heal it with regenerative practices.

Regenerative farming clearly has some way to go yet before it can offer an alternative to current conventional, large-scale agriculture. However, it's equally clear that it is a source of important ideas and influence. For farmers, a regenerative approach can offer new profitable and nature-friendly economic models. For policymakers, it offers alternative ways of thinking about sustainability. And for changemakers looking to reduce the negative impacts of farming, it represents small actions and changes that are closely linked to a large-scale vision.

It implies a general approach that allows for different farms to develop new, adaptive cycles and systems. These, in turn, can support and develop a unique and resilient farm ecosystem. Nature isn't fixed; it's something that involves a co-evolutionary, partnered relationships between human and natural systems.

Probably the biggest challenge to overcome relates to yield. We must continue to feed our growing population whilst regenerating natural systems and ensuring their future productivity. On the surface, industrialized approaches of neat monoculture rows, turbo-charged by chemical inputs, can address both of these needs. What're more industrial methods have proven high yields, and therefore lower land requirements, meaning less expansion into natural land. Green Revolution demonstrated; this way of producing food certainly made plentiful, accessible food possible for most. However, in the long run, this has proved a false economy. More and more chemicals are required to maintain these yields, while at the same time degrading the natural foundation for fertility and abundance — topsoil, biodiversity, and local water systems.

Evidence shows that regenerative approaches can both address environmental and productivity needs. Farms that focus on soil health are experiencing year-on-year yield increases. Examples include Leontino Balbo's Native Farm in Brazil reporting a 20% increase in sugar cane yield; thousands of Indian ZBNF farms measuring boosts in many different crops such as a 36% increase in groundnuts; Takao Furuno's integrated duck-rice model that has led to a 20–50% rice yield increase as well as a tripling in revenue. These are just a few examples that constitute a rapidly growing dataset proving that regenerative approaches can produce sufficient food with higher profit margins.

However, focusing solely on yield would be to fall into the trap of linear thinking. Taking a systemic view leads to systemic benefits: increased resilience, mitigating the health impact of industrial production, and massive reductions in carbon. With so much untapped potential, new commercial opportunities exist in developing new technology and products that make it easier for farmers to practice regenerative agriculture. For example, seed companies could offer specially designed mixes so more farmers could achieve the same benefits.

TENDENCIES AND LINEAGES OF REGENERATIVE AGRICULTURE

Robert Rodale describes the 7 tendencies towards regeneration in agriculture. These seven P's describe how a system moves to being regenerative. It is helpful to understand these seven tendencies as it helps to conceptualize the necessary elements needed to move towards a regenerative agricultural system. What is interesting about this is that Robert also applies these tendencies to regeneration in both communities and personal spirit. Regeneration doesn't exist in a silo, and the benefit for society and the individual shouldn't be neglected.

The first is Pluralism, which essentially means diversity in plant species.

Second, Protection refers to the need for cover crops to end erosion and increase microbial populations near the surface of the soil.

Purity describes the intentional lack of pesticides and fertilizers in production.

The fourth tendency, Permanence calls for more perennials and plants with vigorous roots.

Peace refers to the harmony with nature, growing with it rather than fighting against it.

Potential describes the readily available nutrients that make their way up to the surface of the soil to be used by plants.

The final tendency, Progress, encompasses the ever-improving soil quality in terms of structure and water retention capacity.

LINEAGES OF REGENERATIVE AGRICULTURE

It is important for us to understand that there are various different interpretations of regenerative agriculture. Primarily, we can say that there are 5 primary intellectual and practical lineages of the term "Regenerative Agriculture". Each lineage has a different definition, farming philosophy, and approach relating to that community. It is important to recognize the ethno-centric bias to these lineages as they primarily represent the Anglo-North American perspective. Let's note that for tens of thousands of years, most indigenous peoples on this planet have existed, and some still do, in what might be referred to as a "regenerative" relationship with the natural systems they co-exist with.

1. Rodale Organic

Recall the originator of regenerative agriculture who gave us those 7 Tendencies towards Regeneration? He has been promoting organic farming since the 70s and has just recently rebranded as regenerative. Their main focus is the soil. This lineage claims that "regeneration" is a mix of methods from 40-year-tested conservation farming, including cover-cropping, crop rotation, compost, low or no-till. These are great erosion and input reduction practices, while increasing soil carbon.

2. Permaculture

This lineage of Regenerative Agriculture, along with a heavy emphasis on small-scale design and claims about reversing climate change, tends toward principles from the human potential movement, focusing on how to establish "thriving" and "abundance" for everyone. A lot of successful regenerative farm designs have come out of this lineage, often they effectively integrate agroforestry, comprehensive water-planning, soil-building, and holistic livestock management while building farmer capacity and economic viability.

3. Holistic Management

This lineage is promoted by both the Savory Institute and Holistic Management International. It focuses on a comprehensive decision-making framework designed for animal-centric ecosystem regeneration.

4. Regenerative Paradigm

Charles Krone developed the term 'Regenerative' over 50 years ago to describe a radically different paradigm of approaching the development of humans and systems. It has been instrumental in the construction of the Levels of Regenerative Agriculture which are; Functional, Integrative, Systemic and Evolutionary.

5. Soil Profits / No-Till / NRCS

This lineage, embodied and led by Ray Archuleta, Gabe Brown, and others, draws practices and inspiration from other lineages, but strongly appeals to traditional farmers by avoiding organic farming dogmas and concentrating on bottom line income through improved soil health.

By avoiding the stigma of organic, this approach allows farmers to continue using synthetic inputs while showing the economic arguments for decreasing inputs and improving soil through good crop rotation, no-till, and grazing practices.

CONCLUSION

It's predicted that the world population is set to rise to 9.2 billion by 2050, creating a need for a 60 percent increase in global food production. Currently, 842 million people are undernourished, 827 million of which residing in low-income countries. In low-income countries, spending on food can often consume over half of household income, leaving the poor extremely vulnerable to price fluctuations. Shifts in the system such as climate change, soil degradation, pest outbreaks, economic and political crises, and population growth are placing added pressures on the global food system.

The global food systems are inherently complex, due to their various processes, value chains, actors and interactions. The outcomes of the food system affect multiple stakeholders and industries in various and occasionally conflicting forms. With so many relying on their resilience, food systems must be equipped to meet their goals, even when presented with unpredictable drivers of change.

There are many movements today that are trying to reframe how we produce and consume food. These alternative approaches include agroforestry, permaculture, and others that are founded on the adoption of low external input systems. These approaches are similar in their efforts to close nutrient loops while increasing the fertility of the soil and on-farm biodiversity. However, now we know that these approaches are in fact, not new. Indigenous technology and methods can be exemplified in every single one!

There's a good chance that you've heard about the connection between the COVID-19 Pandemic and conventional agriculture. Industrial farming systems, which have led to the destruction of natural habitats, loss of genetic diversity, and the crowding of animals into factory farms, created vulnerable ecosystems less able to cope with virus outbreaks. Now is as good a time as any to start rethinking how we produce food, before we end up in a never-ending cycle of pandemics and government lockdowns. Our lives depend directly on nature, it's as simple as that. Fortunately, there is much we can do about this.

We are losing topsoil at an alarming rate: last year, the UN warned that with the current level of topsoil depletion, we only have a shocking 60 harvests left. The good news is that we can turn this around. Regenerative Agriculture has the potential to reverse these effects. The purpose of regenerative agriculture is to rebuild soil health by restoring the carbon content in the soil, which positively impacts plant health, nutrition and farm productivity. Regenerative farmers simply work with nature rather than against it.

It all starts and ends with our soil. Healthy soil can absorb more CO2, reducing the amount of carbon in the atmosphere, which will slow down global warming. Also, as soil health improves, its ability to drain water improves as well, allowing underground water aquifers to replenish. This means the soil will naturally protect us from floods and droughts!

In the end, regenerative methods will also have tremendous social benefits. Farmer's livelihoods will be improved through the reduction of costs (artificial inputs/oil-powered equipment), the diverse variety of crops will diversify their offering, and overall, their resilience will be increased. Our health improves when we eat produce grown in healthy soil as those plants will have a higher number of nutrients. A healthy soil biology also protects the roots and the plants itself: in that sense, practicing regenerative agriculture addresses all the usual concerns regarding weeds, pests, droughts, fertility and yield.

Continuous practice of regenerative agricultural system could result in a reduction of up to 22.3 gigatons of carbon dioxide, and an enormous return of financial investments. Even better, converting 298 million hectares of the abandoned degraded farmland globally to regenerative farming or its native vegetation such as forests could lead to the absorption of up to 20.3 gigatons of CO2, with another massive return of financial investment and increased food production.

Sounds amazing right? We think so. The goal is to regenerate 1 million hectares of degraded land by 2030. As we drive to make regenerative agriculture mainstream, the possibilities are endless and we are all in this together.